HYSTERICAL HYSTERECTOMY

MARION HUGHES

HYSTERICAL HYSTERECTOMY

All the characters, events and situations portrayed in this book are factual. In certain instances, names have been changed.

HYSTERICAL HYSTERECTOMY
Copyright © MMXI by Marion Hughes
Marion Hughes has asserted herself as the author of
HYSTERICAL HYSTERECTOMY, an original work.
Cover Design and Book Design by Evonne Hew
© ACASHIC™ INTELLECTUAL CAPITAL PTY LIMITED

All rights reserved including the right to reproduce this book or a portion thereof in any form is strictly prohibited, unless you have contacted the writer to obtain permission.

Published and distributed by

acashic

ACASHIC INTELLECTUAL CAPITAL PTY LIMITED
PO Box 8030, Subiaco East
WA 6008, Australia
+618 9324 4455
mail@acashic.com   acashic@gmail.com

*Font size — 12pt, Cambria   Paper — Book Cream
Editor in Chief: Michael Garcia*

Creative Director & Cover Design: Evonne Hew

Production: Acashic Actuality

Printed in USA

ISBN 978-1-300-68894-5

DISCLAIMER

Acashic Intellectual Capital Pty Limited ("the Publisher") asserts the following in regards to the book ("the Work") and the cover ("the Cover"):

The views expressed on any aspect of the Cover and in the Work are solely those of the Author ("the Author"), other writers and or individuals providing them, and do not reflect the opinions of the Publisher, its parent, affiliate or subsidiary companies. Caution is advised when reading or using the Work. The Publisher is not responsible for any damages sustained by the Reader ("the Reader") or User ("the User") of the Work, when reading or using the Work. The Publisher shall not be responsible for any aspect that may result in claims of defamation and invasion of privacy. In all instances the Publisher has relied on the expertise of the Author and has not investigated the matters provided by the Author. The Publisher has no duty to investigate the factual or other basis of the material provided by the Author.

Protection is deemed to include all of the Publisher's products which includes but is not limited to books, web sites, CD-ROMs, DVDs and other media ("the Products") that give advice or provide instructional information – all of which are protected in their own right under appropriate, legally drafted Disclaimers.

Copying or disseminating any information published by the Publisher, electronic or otherwise is strictly prohibited. The Reader should be aware that the text of the Work is subject to change at any time. Uploading of the Work and its Cover without permission of the Publisher is unauthorized and may lead to a conviction as a result of a piracy suit.

The work is provided by the Publisher on an "as is" basis. The Publisher makes no representations or warranties of any kind, express or implied, as to the operation of the Work, its website(s), the information, content, materials or products, included in the Work. To the full extent permissible by applicable law, the Publisher disclaims all warranties, express or implied, including but not limited to, implied warranties of merchantability and fitness for a particular purpose. The Publisher will not be liable for any damages of any kind arising from the use of the Work, including but not limited to direct, indirect, incidental punitive and consequential damages.

The Authors and the Publisher specifically disclaim any implied warranties of merchantability or fitness for any particular purpose and shall in no event be liable for any loss or profit or other commercial damage, including but not limited to special, incidental, consequential, or other damages incurred as a result of specific decisions made by the Reader and or User.

Publisher does not take responsibility for any Author- or third-party websites or their contents.

It is assumed that a Reader and or User reads books front to back and therefore start at the front flowing through the Disclaimer. This means that the Reader and or the User of the Work has entered into a "contract" with the Publisher that includes that the Reader and or User read and or used the contents and its information in the Work with full knowledge of and agreement with the Disclaimers.

Acting affirmatively or continuing to read and or use the Work is deemed by the Publisher that the Reader and or User accepts the terms and conditions of the Work and or its Disclaimers. If the Reader and or User of the Work refuse to accede to the terms of any of the Disclaimers contained herein, then it is agreed by the Reader and or User that the Reader and or User shall immediately return the Work. If the Reader and or User do not so act, the Publisher may argue that a "contract" was formed with the Reader and or User making the Reader and or User bound by the terms of the Disclaimers.

If the Disclaimers are defective in some way, or that the Disclaimers are defectively placed, the use of all Disclaimers will nevertheless in all instances still act as a claim to a defense.

If a claim, action, or proceeding is brought against the Publisher, its licensees, or any seller of the Work, based on facts which, if true, would violate any of the warranties or representations in this Agreement, Publisher may defend the same through counsel it chooses and may settle the same in its sole discretion.

Copyright © MMX Acashic Intellectual Capital Pty Ltd. No portion of the Work including its Disclaimers may be copied, transmitted, retransmitted, posted, reposted, duplicated or otherwise used without the express written approval of the Publisher.

AUTHOR'S DISCLAIMER

The Authors assert the following in regards to the book ("the Work") and the cover ("the Cover"):

Caution is advised when reading or using the Work. The Authors are not responsible for any damages sustained by the Reader ("the Reader") or User ("the User") of the Work, when reading or using the Work. The Authors shall not be responsible for any aspect that may result in claims of defamation and invasion of privacy. In all instances, and as far as is reasonably possible, the Authors have relied on third party representations and expertise.

It is assumed that a Reader and or User reads books front to back and therefore start at the front flowing through the Disclaimer. This means that the Reader and or the User of the Work has entered into a "contract" with the Author that includes that the Reader and or User read and or used the contents and its information in the Work with full knowledge of and agreement with the Disclaimers.

Acting affirmatively or continuing to read and or use the Work is deemed by the Author that the Reader and or User accepts the terms and conditions of the Work and or its Disclaimers. If the Reader and or User of the Work refuse to accede to the terms of any of the Disclaimers contained herein, then it is agreed by the Reader and or User that the Reader and or User shall immediately return the Work. If the Reader and or User do not so act, the Author may argue that a "contract" was formed with the Reader and or User making the Reader and or User bound by the terms of the Disclaimers.

If the Disclaimers are defective in some way, or that the Disclaimers are defectively placed, the use of all Disclaimers will nevertheless in all instances still act as a claim to a defense.

If a claim, action, or proceeding is brought against the Authors, its licensees, or any seller of the Work, based on facts which, if true, would violate any of the warranties or representations in this Agreement, the Authors may defend the same through counsel it chooses and may settle the same in their sole discretion.

ACKNOWLEDGEMENTS

After my hysterectomy, I decided to write this book for all women who are, or might be thinking of undergoing the procedure or who know family or friends who may be too.

To my ever patient, ever loving husband, Dave (Hughesy), always there, always supporting me in whatever I do, and trust me there has been some classics, my soul mate, my best friend.

Sheriden Amanda, my precious daughter, we have been through so much and I adore her with a passion beyond words.

My boys, Louis and Max, the best two boys a mother could ever have.

Loving, caring, funny and clever...a pleasure always; I love them to bits (that doesn't get you out of emptying the dishwasher, boys!)

I love you all so much it hurts.

I am proud to be your mum.

My Dad (Ted) would not be where I am without him, he got me through so much and is always there for us, love you dad.

My brother Brian and his family, thanks just for being you and enriching our lives.

My family are my life.

What surrounds me is an added bonus.

I have special friends and acquaintances who balance a "just about perfect" life.

Everyday I wake up is a good day.

When I close my eyes at night with us all under the same roof there is nothing more that I need.

Remember:

What doesn't kill you makes you stronger.

CONTENTS

1
What Should You Pack? **12**

2
What Happens After Surgery? **17**

3
What You Can Do At Home? **26**

4
What Else? **34**

5
Top 5 Dos And Don'ts? **46**

WHY IS IT ESSENTIAL READING?

This surgery is by no means a pleasant experience but I can guarantee there is not one lady involved in the procedure that will not benefit from these words of wisdom and humour, a bible in do's and don'ts that can save unnecessary pain, depression and possibly more surgery.

Essential reading, Hysterical Hysterectomy will make the whole procedure a safer more enjoyable experience.

Oh, how I wish that I had this book before I went into hospital for my hysterectomy! We are talking major surgery here.

Go ahead google Hysterectomy and you will most likely only find how to correctly spell the word, absolutely nothing informative.

Calling various organisations, getting the same answer, "Just be careful." "So what is careful?" I asked, at which point it all went quiet, "Just careful, lovey."

Right I thought adjusting my cushions bring it on, so precariously balanced I started to share my story in a very informative and light hearted manner.

Knowledge in this situation is like gold, major surgery should automatically demand extensive literature, but in this case sadly not.

To share my experience and greatly benefit from yours share what you learn and contact me within at *acashic@acashic.com.*

Hysterically Yours,
MARION HUGHES

INTRODUCTION

I decided after my hysterectomy to write this for you.

After returning home I made many calls and researched on the net, but nothing was really of any help in helping me compile this book.

"Just be sensible."

What exactly is sensible? I have three children, a husband and a house to run.

"Just don't lift anything heavier than a litre, love, and you will be fine."

Well, that was a great help. (Not!)

My one "hysterectomy information pamphlet" hung precariously on a fridge magnet, its content as helpful as the magnet that held it.

...So, girls... hang on to yer knickers (literally).

Please note any medical terms or advice are from my own experience, although totally relevant. They are not to be strictly relied on, please seek medical advice if you are unsure.

❋❦❋

I was going to end the book with this paragraph but I believe in telling it as it is, and if I was to lie, then what kind of mate would I be? It is a big operation and sometimes ignorance can be bliss, but when the benefits far outweigh the negatives then go girl, you have so got the power to get through and come out a stronger fitter woman. Like childbirth the pain is soon forgotten, and the benefits start to shine, ask those questions even if they seem silly, it's your body sweetheart and you won't be asking anything that hasn't been asked before.

It really isn't that bad, I just love writing a story. If anything I have written helps you just a bit, then it will be worth it, stay strong and keep this little book by your side.

1

What Should You Pack?

Firstly a few tips for the hospital.

When packing, think of everything within reason:

- ✓ **A HAIRDRYER**, and not for the hair on your head, it dries your undercarriage with ease and efficiency, no rubbing just warm air, aahhh!! Don't knock it 'til you try it.

- ✓ **ANTIBACTERIAL WIPES**, it is almost impossible to dangle in your delicate state, and sitting on a toilet seat where a complete stranger has been is not my cup of tea, especially with more than usual bodily fluids present. As clean as hospitals are, it is impossible to police those toilets all the time. If you are lucky enough to be a private patient, then ensure your visitors refrain from using your facility.

- **CHANGE FOR THE PHONE**, and important phone numbers.

- **BOOKS** (including this one) and magazines.

- **SANITARY PADS** of the surfboard variety, you will be glad of the padding.

- **SENSIBLE KNICKERS**

- **SENSIBLE NIGHTIES**, ones that go to your knees, and a dressing gown.

- **A BED-JACKET** or cardigan.

- **DEFIANTLY SLIP-ON SLIPPERS** that slip on without having to bend down.

- **EARPLUGS** if not guaranteed own room.

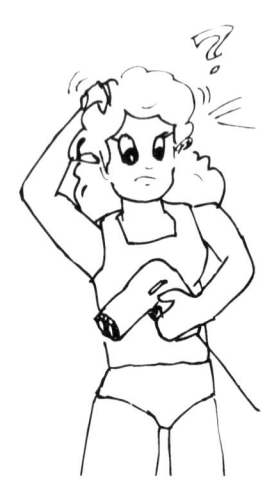

Pack a hairdryer

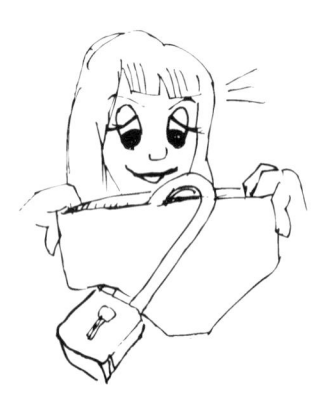

Wear sensible knickers

✓ **TREAT YOURSELF TO NICE SMELLIES** for your shower care.

✓ **MOISTURISER**, the conditions and surgery will take it out. Keep "nice and moist", if you know what I mean.

✓ **COUGH SWEETS**, the constant air-conditioned environment caused me to get an annoying dry cough — the cough sweets were magic.

✓ **A FEW NIBBLES** or treats are nice to have on hand.

Be in control and ask questions, not just with the doctor but the anaesthetist and nurses.

From experience I know I turn into a vomatron after anaesthetics, and the medication "to stop me being sick" makes me sick.

Because I got the right dose, I was fine.

Only take essential items to the actual shower with you, you will be surprised how heavy that wash bag can get — especially if *I* am packing it.

The lady opposite me had her husband there most of the time, and the girl next to me had many male visitors.

Don't be shy about keeping your curtains closed, getting in and out of bed in a lady-like manner is no mean feat.

I was dying for a wee one night, but knew my nightie would not cover my essentials, the curtains were open and there were a lot of visitors in the room.

Just ask the nurse to keep them closed, it's your right to feel comfortable.

2

What Happens After Surgery?

OK, SO I AM HAVING A HYSTERECTOMY; "the best thing you could ever do," said all those that had had it done. What they didn't tell me was that it felt like a Mac truck had driven up my fanny, done a 3 point turn, dropped its load skidded a few times then reversed out sideways on, then a staple gun was used to repair any damage.

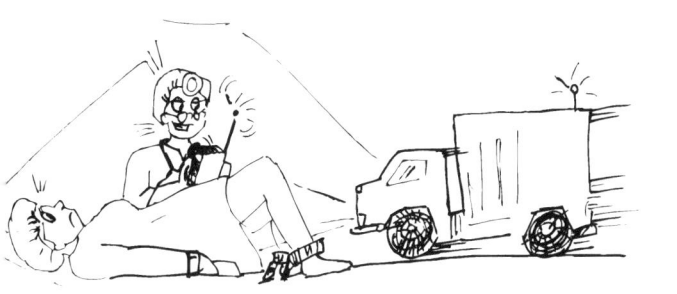

Waking up attached to a multitude of tubes, bottles and bags you soon realise any dignity you preserved from having your children has been left in the car park on the way in. This procedure always reminds me of the joke about the gynaecologist who wallpapered his hallway through the letterbox.

Of course if the procedure was done through open surgery, and not vaginally then the Mac truck entered that way, did its duty then reversed out, same difference, only your precious undercarriage remains intact, and hardly aware of what's gone on a few inches up.

To be honest. At first the pain wasn't really too bad, but the pump-control pain-relief soon became my best friend and when I heard the nurse say she was removing it, I pressed it to buggery, ensuring every last drop entered my veins before it was whipped heartlessly away.

I lay there thinking what have I done as the lady in the next bed vomited with such high volume it sounded like a loudhailer had been used instead of a sick bowl. She then

HYSTERICAL HYSTERECTOMY

proceeded to groan in the same manner, and then snore like a dying buffalo for the rest of the night. Lovely jubbly!

No amount of pillows on my head could take away that wall-shaking noise. As soon as morning came, I sneaked my contraband mobile out from under the sheets and messaged my husband. SOD THE FLOWERS! JUST BRING ME SOME BLOODY EAR PLUGS! That he did. Just as well, because the other two women in the room decided to make it a concerto that night. I was just nodding off in time to be woken by the nurse to give me a sleeping tablet.

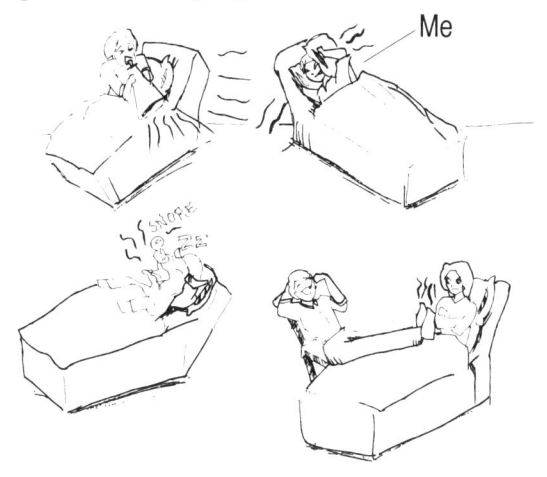

The next day they decided to get me vertical. When the colour of my face matched the sheets they soon realised that my request to leave it a few hours was a valid one, and off they trotted.

Later that day we tried again and made a triumphant stroll to the door and back — all of 3 metres — but a triumph no less.

Back to bed and, roll on, brekkie.

Having had soup and jelly for tea the night before, I was looking forward to breakfast, which basically was the same, in fact I am convinced — the very same.

Lunch wasn't much better.

This light-diet thing was no fun, but trapped by the multitude of tubes, I had no choice but to conform.

DAY TWO was basically confined to bed with little trips to the door and back.

DAY THREE arrives; oh joy, I get to go to the loo, that joy was also short lived when I was presented with a bowl and jug.

"Just wee into that, love, and tip it into the jug and measure it."

Ok, so let's waddle with the catheter bag in one hand and jug and bowl in the other — so where do I put my spare pad, under my chin maybe?

That short trip to the loos was an eternity

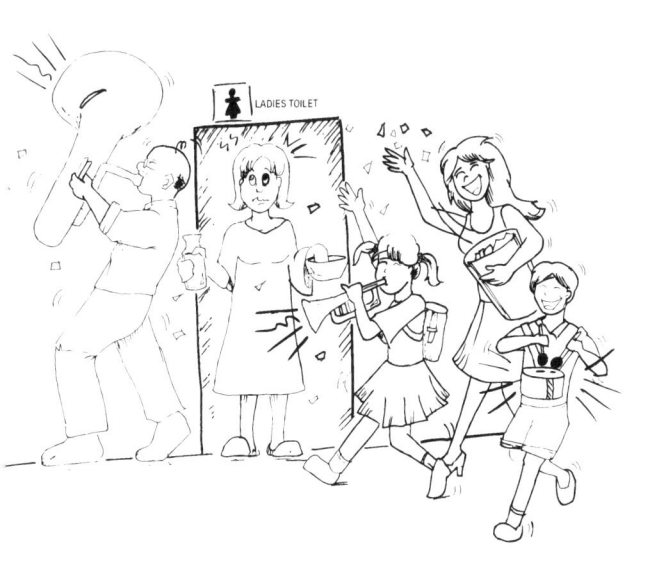

with what seemed like the whole household cavalry passing by just at that very time, husbands and grandfathers and inquisitive children. *Oh do beam me up Scotty* thought.

After tackling that God-forsaken procedure, I had to return the same journey, only this time saying "200ml" over and over in my mind, worried that my anaesthetically-poisoned mind would forget it, and I would have to start from scratch.

After that, I was told I would have to do the same again all day, this time turning off the catheter tube, in between wees to see if I emptied my bladder.

Now, here's a tip, listen to what you are told. Wee, then wait a few minutes, lean forward and back, then wee again. It's called "voiding".

This I did, and totally flummoxed the nurses as they ultra-sounded to find no wee present in my bladder at all.

After weeing, catching it in the trusty bowl then measuring it, I repeated the procedure for 24 hours.

This I did successfully, with each changing shift — amazed that I managed to totally remove any water from my bladder.

The idea is to ensure your bladder is in working-order before the removal of the catheter.

After that was removed I felt like skipping to my loo, but the waddle was still the way to go. That Mac truck had sure made an impression.

Just a private word...

If you are fortunate enough to have private cover, the previous few tasks will be a more relaxing experience, as the trip to the toilet should be shorter and with much less passing traffic in a private hospital. I think my experience was not indicative of most, as the hospital was pre-war with mixed wards and shared rooms — anyway, I digress again.

DAY FOUR Ok, "one more night of the buffalo concerto and I'm out of here." Earplugs adorned, I skulled my fibre gel in anticipation of my final task. The night nurse was well aware of my eagerness to be discharged and I asked her to put in a good word.

"Everything working and functioning ok?" my gynaecologist asked on his morning rounds.

"Absolutely," I said, crossing my fingers under the covers, "Can I go home?"

The word "yes" was music to my ears; the other music (of the wind variety) was as a result of the surgery, just as well the sheets were tucked in tightly, otherwise the lady in the opposite bed would have been wearing them.

This is the only time I have got away with farting like a Docker; with not being allowed to strain it's amazing how something can slip out so loud, anyway I digress again.

As the doctor disappeared again, down the corridor a little face appeared from behind the curtain.

"You haven't had a poo yet, have you?"

I couldn't lie, "Well, he didn't specifically say, 'have you pooed' so I didn't specifically answer."

With that, she returned five minutes later and politely asked me to roll over.

HYSTERICAL HYSTERECTOMY

Just think of England I thought as she deposited the suppository where the sun don't shine.

Now I knew my husband would be here any time, and my only ticket out was to go to the toilet.

Should I lie or not?

Just as I was considering it, the suppositories decided for me, well that's a load off my mind, let's get out of here.

Leaving the other three women in their beds wishing they had been as regimented as me, I scooted as fast as my Mac-damaged vagina would carry me.

The car journey home was less than comfortable; it felt like the whole of the highway had been fitted with speed bumps at 10 metre-intervals.

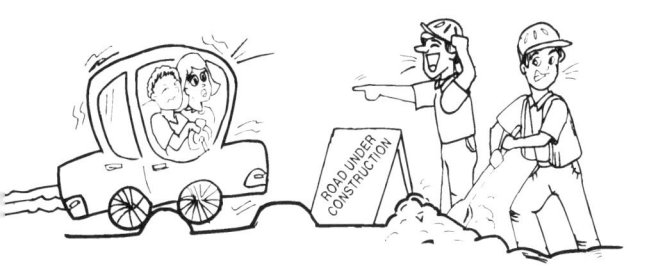

3

What You Can Do At Home?

Great to be home to my own loo and bed.

Every cushion and pillow had been seconded until I was perched in a comfortable position to resume 2 weeks of doing virtually nothing.

And this, my loves, is where the 'what can I do now?' came in.

All the books and nurses say, "Just be sensible." I have never had a hysterectomy so what exactly is sensible? All it basically told me was: don't pick up anything heavier than a one litre jug and no pushing or pulling movements; gradually increase your exercise and activities, but don't open any large heavy

HYSTERICAL HYSTERECTOMY

swinging doors (just as well I decided not to get them for my bedroom, I thought).

Now what?

My gyno said don't drive for 6 weeks — my little booklet said drive after 2 if you feel comfortable. The stories are so conflicting I decided to write a more precise do's and don'ts. Now I am not a doctor, but few personal experiences are always a good thing to have.

Take no notice of Gertrude next door who's had every near death operation since childbirth. She will scare the bejabers out of you; with her stories of being lacerated from end to end and stitched with fishing wire; always hobbling and sick but she will trample over you to get to the last piece of cream cake, or will run the length of the driveway to nag the postie for riding over her prize petunias.

Now while you can laugh about it after, it's no fun worrying about splitting stitches or worse, I trotted precariously off to my doctors with my list of can I do's, he helped a bit, but it's still a worry. So here we go.

FOR THE FIRST 2 WEEKS

✓ Don't lift anything heavier than a litre jug, that includes children. They will have to be happy with a special "sitting-down" hug.

✓ Do rest as often as you can. You have had major surgery. Do not underestimate it; or over estimate your capabilities.

✓ When rising from a chair or bed, roll out, as opposed to directly lifting yourself up; this will lessen trauma and pulling to your multitude of hidden stitches.

✓ Do not shower by yourself. Make sure someone is in the house. Don't be ashamed to ask for help.

✓ Each day take a short walk. The mail box and back. Maybe a couple of circuits of the back garden. Gradually increase the distance, day by day. Remember by going street-walking you may feel uncomfortable, but still have to make the journey home. By

HYSTERICAL HYSTERECTOMY

walking around the garden, if you start to feel like it's too much, the back door will be looking good.

✔ Having a warm salt bath is great. The bath should only be a few inches deep, so that no water is allowed to enter the vagina so as to cause a possible infection. One thing I found comforting was to saturate a pad in warm salted water and then sit on it — of course with the aid of towels. This saved me from having to negotiate a bath when movements are not your friend. You can shove the pads in a plastic bag and into the fridge or freezer, one of them in yer knickers, helps to numb the pain.

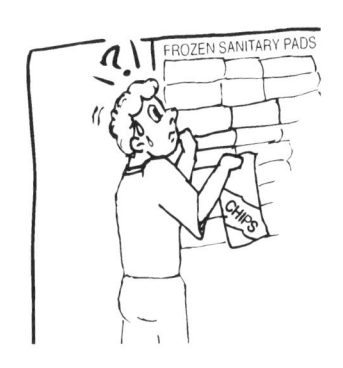

Keep frozen sanitary pads handy

Going back to the pads again, as the bleeding should not be too heavy, those fatter pads (surf boards) given to you in the hospital may not seem necessary, but I (the normal user of g-string pads) actually kept on using them as I found they provided extra cushioning and comfort when sitting or walking.

I was unable to have anyone at home with me, so I made a list of things I would need that day, my husband or daughter would put some milk in a separate jug, so I would not have to lift the full 2 litres (1 litre over the allowed limit).They made my lunch easily accessible either in the fridge or on the work top, and anything I needed for that day was close to hand. The remote control always being top of that list.

Before going into hospital I made curries etc., and froze them, also Lennard's and such shops were very handy. I bought schnitzels, Kiev's and other such goodies, that only required a stint in the oven, a salad and maybe a jacket spud while the chicken is cooking.

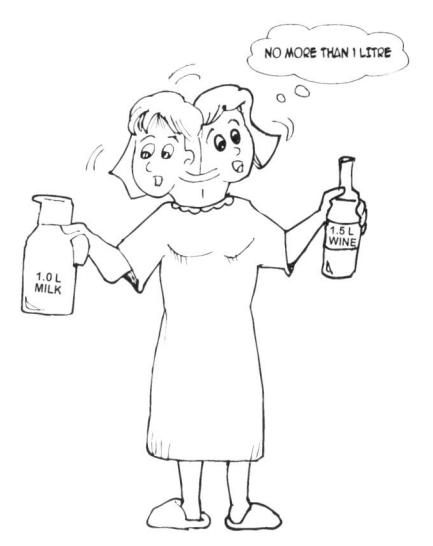

This took the pressure off everyone who had either had a full day at school or work. This can obviously be changed to suit your family's needs, but you get the idea. I am one of these annoying people that have everything sorted down to the last lettuce leaf, but it certainly made life easier.

- **RESTING** Most importantly, don't feel bad about just laying around, you really have to do it. One thing I did do to feel more human, was to insist that I was washed and dressed out of my pj's before 10am; it does make a difference, believe me. It makes the difference between day and night seem more acceptable, and being in the same clothing for 24 hours has other disadvantages.

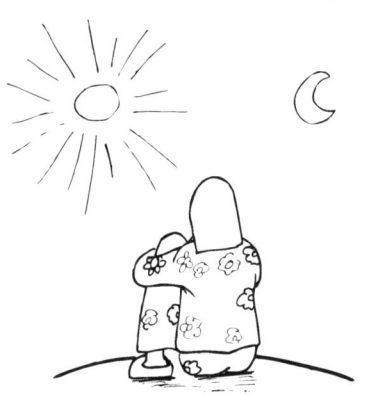

✓ **INFLATABLE RUBBER RING** I invested in a blow-up rubber ring, after trying to balance my dinner on my slanted lap, I felt much more civilised sitting up to the table with the rest of the family, quickly returning to crash position, before the last mouthful fully reached my stomach.

HYSTERICAL HYSTERECTOMY

- **TOILET TRIPS** Talking of the stomach and the resulting movements or not, do drink plenty of water and take fibre-gel or something similar. Remember you are not allowed to strain at all, and as yucky as this sounds you do have to work it down and sit for a while awaiting the next performance. As the song goes don't push it don't force it, let it happen naturally. I think this is very important to remember.

- **STRETCHING** Another very important one is not to stretch high. If there is something that you need up there too bad. You have been such a good girl, why blow it and the stitches? I was concerned about using the hair dryer and lifting my arms up. For the first 3 weeks I placed the hairdryer on a towel on the bed and sat in front of it, and just styled the best I could.

- **TAKING NAPS** Always make sure you allow yourself the privilege of an extra 1-2 hour nap, you will feel the benefit.

4

What Else?

THE NEXT 3 TO 4 WEEKS

Now don't get too cocky; the worst is over and normal life can resume very slowly? With a big emphasise on slowly, you still need to rest. I did allow myself to peel vegies, and wipe the work top down very gently, I think I even cleaned the loos, and this is where the sensible part comes in. Peel the vegies and leave them in water, don't be tempted to go for the saucepan, and certainly don't lift anything that will cause you damage. I must say I did graduate past a 1 litre jug in my fourth week. That was only because my husband forgot to fill my little jug. With great trepidation I managed it, and felt no ill-effects, but that doesn't make it ok. Just be wary that a little too much confidence could put you back to step one, and that my loves will never do.

✓ **DRIVING** As far as driving goes there lies the conflict. At this point I would exercise much caution, as you will be truly amazed how many muscles you do use to drive, so here I will give you my story but you must be very careful. My gyno is a lovely man who tends to side with caution, which is great if you have a big support team around you to drive the kids to school. His 6 week demand was too much for me to bear. My own GP and the all of one pamphlet that I had, suggested two weeks but only if you feel comfortable in the seat buckled up. If you have an automatic with power-steering then that makes a lot of difference too, I would not be so quick to risk a manual or non-power-steering, and the jury is still out on that one. Me personally, I started mid my third week. Just to our local shops which is a two km round journey. And then only when I felt 100% sure I felt alright did I made the journey to school which is a twenty two km round trip, and that's my lot. No out of town journeys just because you feel it's ok. Stay within a certain limit, after you graduate the six weeks — go girl!

✓ **MENIAL HOUSEWORK** Ignore the ten layers of dust that have accumulated, or do what I did so as not to feel completely useless. I bought one of those Pledge grab-it gadgets that allow you to dust with absolutely no effort at all, that's of course if you feel the need. It also passes the time and does somehow make you feel like you have accomplished something. It was totally doing my head in watching the television with each of my kids names aimlessly etched on the top of the box, one swipe and it was gone, a result, a small one but a result no less.

✓ **GET HELP** Just hang on in there nothing is more important than you at the moment. If your hubby tends not to be on the helpful side, then maybe take him along to a doctor's

HYSTERICAL HYSTERECTOMY

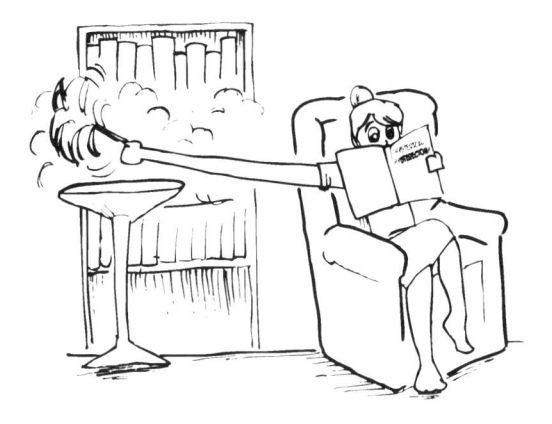

visit or give him the one pamphlet you were given. It most certainly won't hurt the children to be more accommodating either. If you are by yourself then get help — it is available; ask your doctor before you leave hospital.

- **SEX** Talking of husbands, partners or whatever you happen to have at the time, there is one subject we have not approached and that's sex, yes sex. Just like the poo thing it is something that the doctors prefer you can do to make sure all is well.

Be in control, lovely lady, relaxation and lubrication. How, when, where; take it slow, very slow. It all still works fine, it's just had a few adjustments, like the Mac truck doing a three point turn and skidding out. Believe me, it's in their interests to listen to you. If it doesn't feel right, then leave it and if frustration prevails then another form of relief may have to take place, if you get my drift. It is best to do the deed, after the six weeks — unless informed otherwise.

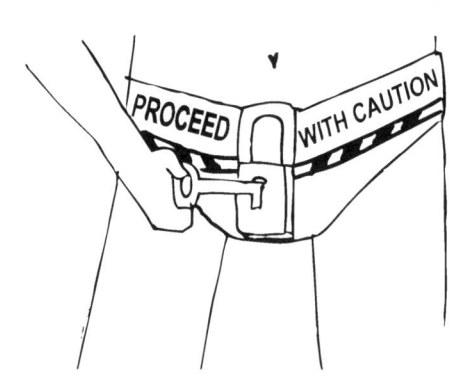

When it comes to sex

This basically concludes the requirements for you to return to normal duties.

Now we have been there, done that, I feel comfortable enough to tell you not to panic if there is a small amount of blood after the performance, or if it was very uncomfortable, let your specialist know and he will examine you. This is very common and it just basically means you need a little help to get the vagina there I said it vagina, vagina, vagina. It's one of those words, eh? (I will tell you a funny story in a minute) anyway I digress again. It all needs a little stretch and this is done by the use of a strange object made of glass that you insert and leave there for an allotted time. It does not hurt but it helps immensely. I sneezed one night after inserting it and it flew out across the room. My husband's diving-catch was worthy of a place in the England team. The look on his face was priceless when he realised what he was holding.

Now mine was hired, yes, hired would you believe like a DVD, with a deposit returned on completion. Now this is my story. Other doctor's states or countries may have different methods, so just go with it.

Now my vagina story.

*I was in the shops with my then   year old and he was asking what was for dinner I told him lasagne   Now where this next comment came from I do not know   At the top of his voice he shouted   Yes   Vagina for tea
sure whether I was embarrassed or in total shock   but with the whole shop looking at me I calmly said   Oh yes   and we all know dad likes seconds of that*

Talking of stories I could go on forever, but here is another. Shopping for sensible knickers before surgery I was in one of my 'anything could happen' moods,

There just happened to be a sale on and there were women grabbing undies like crazy   as one lady walked away with an armful she dropped some   so full of mischief I grabbed the nearby microphone and announced there is a lady that has dropped her knickers in aisle one   then I could not contain myself and announced clean up in aisle   and

Back to the serious stuff now

HYSTERICAL HYSTERECTOMY

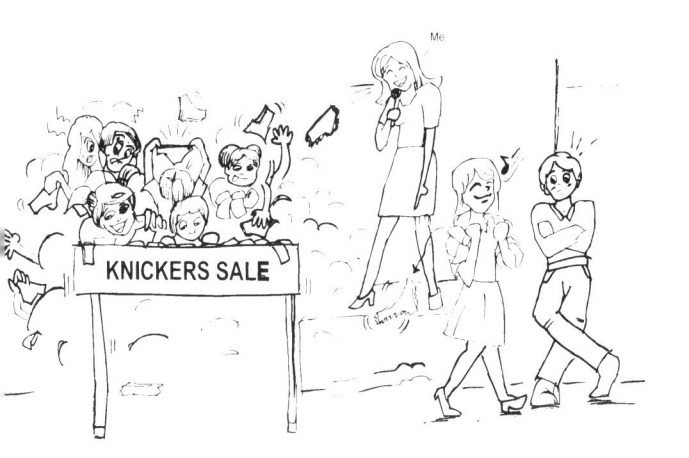

The knickers sale

I can't emphasise more how important it is not to be complacent. If I have to scare you then I will. Nasty things can happen like ovaries (if you decide or can keep them) sticking to bowels or other nasty complications that will require more surgery, which could mean colostomy bags and other such niceties. The lady in the next bed to me was in for more surgery because she was naughty and did too much too soon. She had to come in for corrective surgery, which basically put her back to square one.

So please, please be a good girl, and like me it will all work out, the perfect result and life is good.

✓ **EMOTIONS** will run high, you have been through major surgery, and because there is nothing visible apart from walking like you have just got off the Melbourne cup winner, don't ever underestimate your feelings.

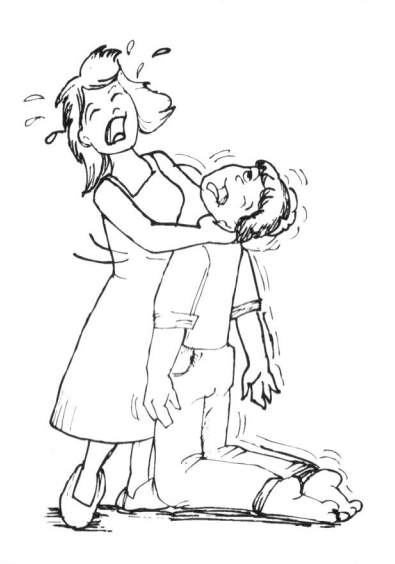

Where are my evening primrose tablets

✓ **SIDE EFFECTS** I basically took it in my stride, and just figured, "Well, it's done, and I am going to be all the better for it."

I, however, kept my ovaries, and did not experience the possible effects of menopause.

There are so many alternatives on the market now to help with these symptoms, so please do not accept the first one.

If you are getting adverse affects, some women get great relief from natural alternatives.

Again, it is your body, and your state of mind.

Find a doctor that sympathises and is prepared to treat you with the respect you deserve.

If, like me, you kept your ovaries, then still be mindful of your condition.

Feeling like you want to do something nasty to your partner is not natural although common, so a visit to your trusty doctor will help to get you through this stage.

✓ **PAP SMEARS** Now most doctors say you will not need this procedure anymore, as you do not have a cervix, but it may be that conditions in the past such as abnormal pap smear results or vaginal worts, etc. will still require the test to be done.

To ensure this most delicate area remains trouble free, the procedure is called a vault smear.

Forget thoughts of flying through the air on the end of a pole, it is as before, just a different name, but still as important.

Soon you will be feeling fantastic, and know more about "which muscle does what", than you ever learned in your biology classes — as you have spent the last six weeks realising that; just reaching for the remote control, uses more stomach muscles than you thought you had in your whole body.

✓ **NOW A BIT FOR THE PARTNERS OR HUSBANDS,** so please get them to read it, it may help.

HYSTERICAL HYSTERECTOMY

Now then   your lovely lady has just had major surgery   please   please   please   do n underestimate her needs

Disobeying the rules could put her back in hospital for more surgery.

Things have been moved, and tampered with; they need time to settle back into the place they were born into.

They don't say 6 weeks for nothing.

We are talking big stuff here, and in order to make a full recovery total T.L.C. (TOTAL LOVING CARE) will be required.

Getting out of a chair will be like climbing Mount Everest

Using the toilet and bath   equally challenging

Keep all she needs within reach   including you   if you can

If not   then keep everything needed for the day within easy reach

No driving for a minimum of   weeks each doctor will have their own take on that

but   always   listen to them

5

Top 5 Dos And Don'ts?

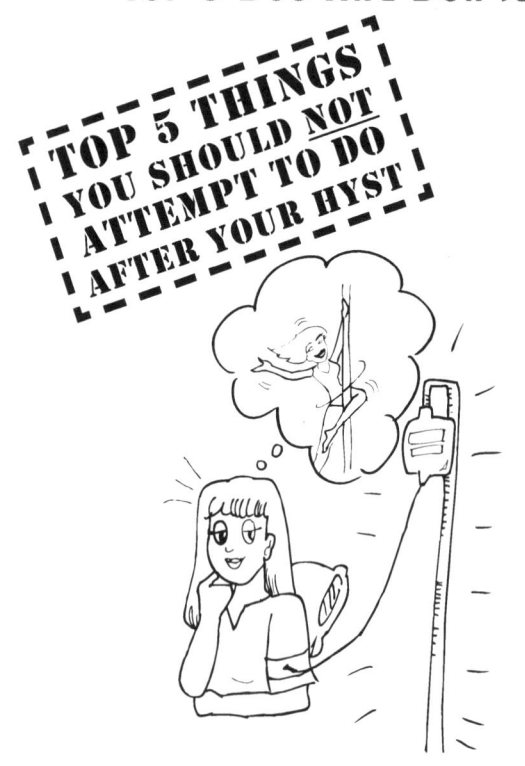

TOP 5 THINGS YOU SHOULD NOT ATTEMPT TO DO AFTER YOUR HYST

DO NOT join a pole dancing club

HYSTERICAL HYSTERECTOMY

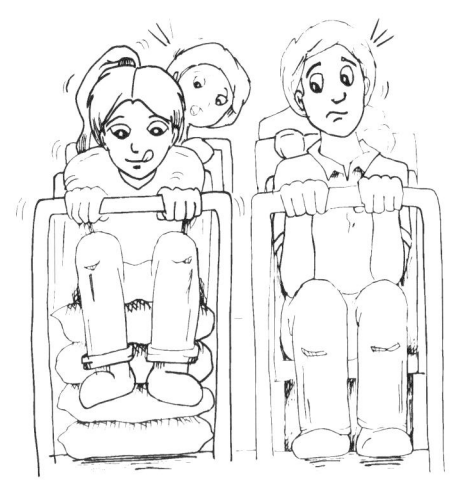

DO NOT take a trip to a theme park

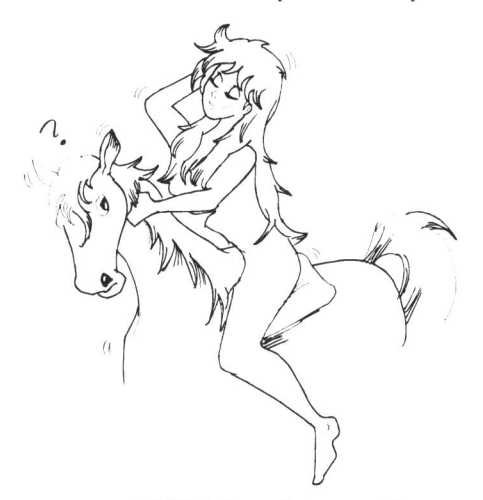

DO NOT do nude horse riding

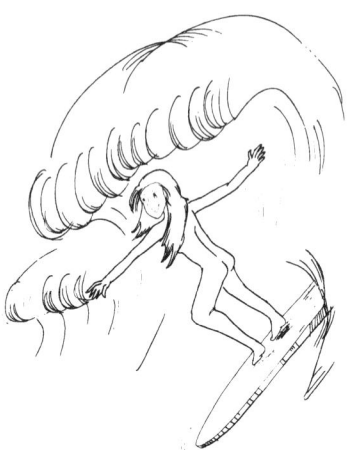

OR anything nude for that matter

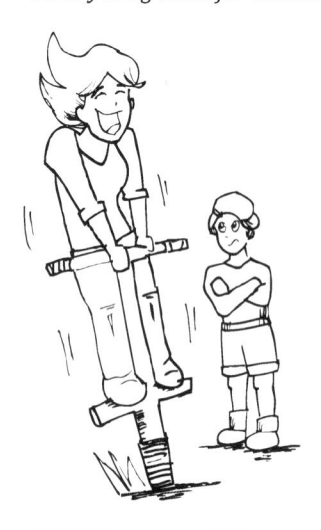

DO NOT try out a kid‍'s pogo stick

HYSTERICAL HYSTERECTOMY

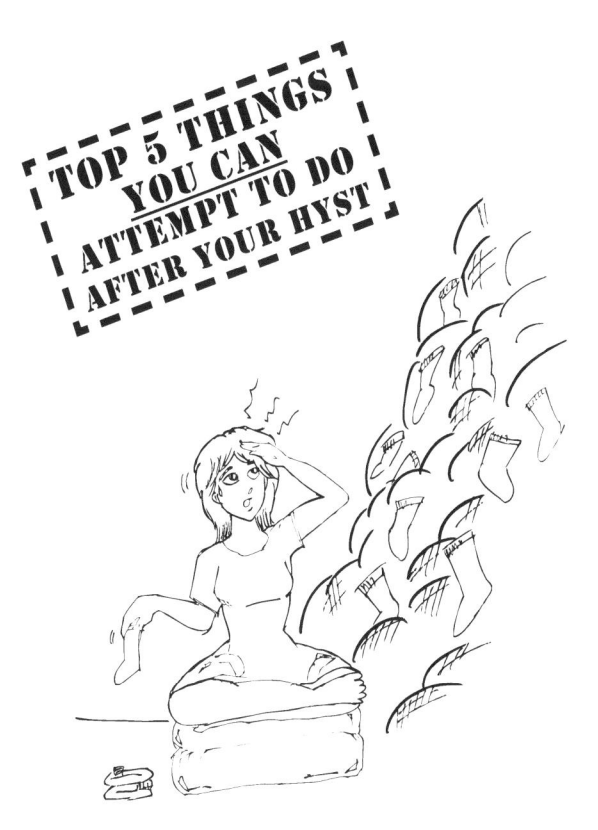

TOP 5 THINGS YOU CAN ATTEMPT TO DO AFTER YOUR HYST

DO sort out the odd sock mountain
no excuses you've got the time

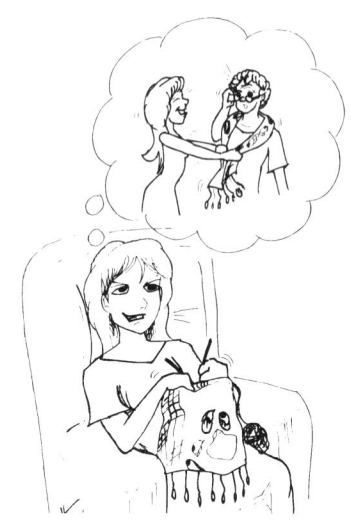

*DO knit scarfs for all the family
get back at Nanna with a tragic jumper
and make her wear it all Christmas day*

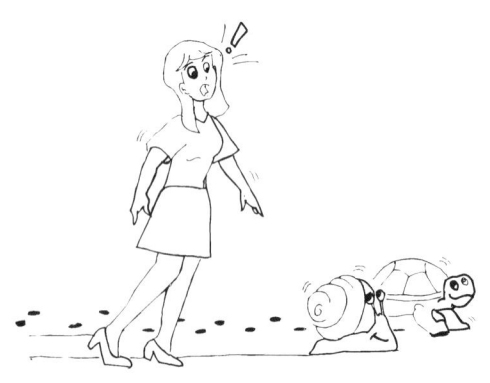

*DO slow walks to the mail box
gradually building up over days*

HYSTERICAL HYSTERECTOMY

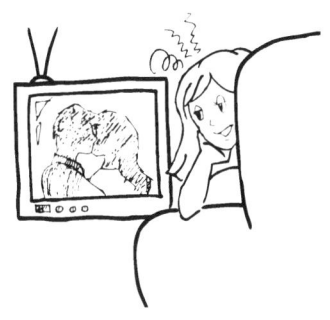

DO watch every crap soap that ever existed on daytime television   just because you can

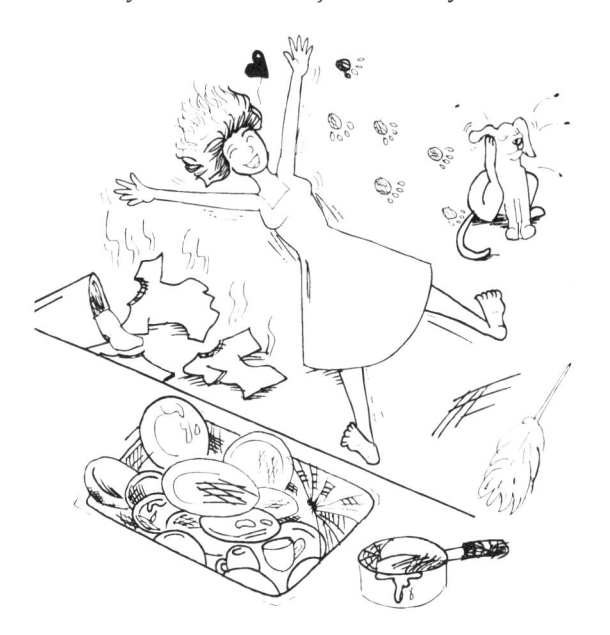

DO learn to love dust and dirty dishes

Well, girls, I hope this has been of assistance and brought a smile to your face.

Look after yourself and do not be afraid to ask even the silliest of questions. You are important and don't forget it. This is major surgery and should not be taken lightly.

Be strong and in control, my dear. You are special and don't you forget it.

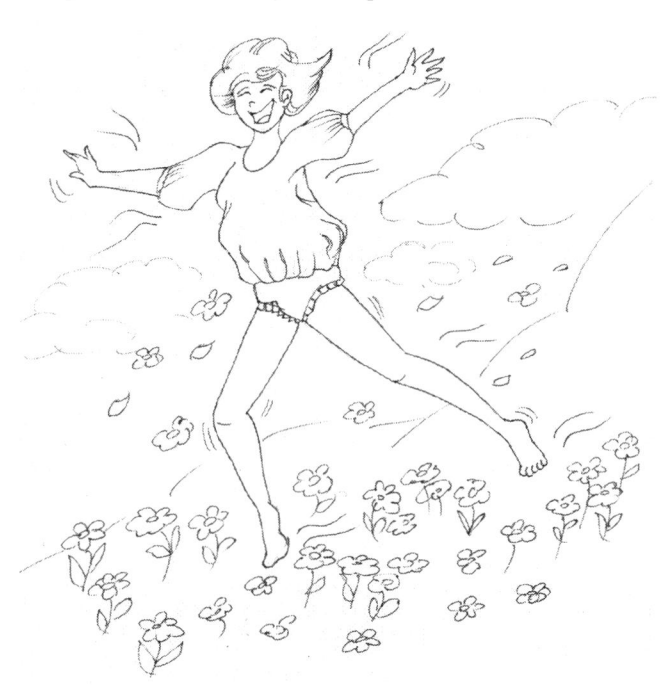

Printed in Great Britain
by Amazon